LEAN AND GREEN

DIET COOKBOOK

FOR BEGINNERS

21 Day Fueling Hacks & Lean and Green Recipes to Help You to Achieve a Life-long Transformation With 5 & 1 and 4 & 2 & 1 Meal Plan

Diamond Connors – DC PRESS

The content and information contained in this book has been compiled from sources deemed reliable, and it is accurate to the best of the Author's knowledge, information and belief. However, the Author cannot guarantee its accuracy and validity and cannot be held liable for any errors and/or omissions. Further, changes are periodically made to this book as and when needed. Where appropriate and/or necessary, you must consult a professional (including but not limited to your doctor, attorney, financial advisor or such other professional advisor) before using any of the suggested remedies, techniques, or information in this book.

Upon using the contents and information contained in this book, you agree to hold harmless the Author from and against any damages, costs, and expenses, including any legal fees potentially resulting from the application of any of the information provided by this book. This disclaimer applies to any loss, damages or injury caused by the use and application, whether directly or indirectly, of any advice or information presented, whether for breach of contract, tort, negligence, personal injury, criminal intent, or under any other cause of action.

You agree to accept all risks of using the information presented inside this book.

You agree that by continuing to read this book, where appropriate and/or necessary, you shall consult a professional (including but not limited to your doctor, attorney, or financial advisor or such other advisor as needed) before using any of the suggested remedies, techniques, or information in this book.

The need for a convenient meal replacement diet has seen a massive surge in recent times for its effective weight loss approach. One such famous and effective meal replacement diet is known as the Lean & Green Diet. The Lean & Green Diet is primarily based on having lean & green meals with consuming small portions throughout the day along with special fuelings. The Lean & Green diet includes specialfood categories that include pre-packaged foods, bar, and shakes, etc. which are also known as "fuelings". The Lean & Green Diet primarily focuses on an effective weight loss approach by eating small portions of food throughout the day to meet your body requirements.

There are two prominent plans in the Lean & Green Diet, i.e., the 5 & 1 plan and the 4 & 2 & 1 plan. The prior is considered optimal for those people who want to achieve a very drastic and rapid weight loss by only consuming 800 calories per day. Whereas the latter is for those people who want to have a relatively slower weight loss or if they want to maintain their current weight. The Lean & Green Diet utmost convenience, clarity in food choices, and rapid weight loss to its followers.

The basic concept of a lean and green diet is to eat portion-controlled high-protein and low carb meals and snacks, known as "Lean and green meals," that we can cook by ourselves, combined with special food categories like *pre-packaged foods, bars, and shakes, known as "Fuelings."*

The lean and green diet is one of the most nutritious regimens out there. It's meant to be more environmentally friendly than other programs like veganism and vegetarianism, but still, provides good nutrition for your body. The principle behind this diet is to focus on whole foods that have minimal processing (they are raw or cooked at low temperatures) and avoid foods with a lot of chemicals.

This diet makes you feel good both physically and mentally as it promotes health in a nontoxic way. People who have the time and resources should follow this regimen. Like with any diet, it requires a significant amount of time and willpower. If you have the chance to do some home cooking or would rather not shop in supermarkets that sell processed foods, this is an excellent way to live a healthy lifestyle. You could also try it merely as a change in some aspects of your everyday life, or as an addition to other diets if you are on a restricted budget.

Lean and green is a program that involves a combination of fresh and pre-prepared foods and snacks. It also offers additional help from a designated support person. Once you have completed your 12-week start-up plan, your average lean and green meal should then include 5–7 ounces of cooked lean protein, plus 3 servings of non-starchy vegetables, and up to 2 servings of healthy fats. The plan is to eat up to 6 meals throughout the day.

If you wish to lose more weight than you lose in the first phase, you can stay on the initial diet plan longer, until you reach your target weight. Once you have reached that weight,

*you should safely enter the "Transition phase."
This involves slowly increasing your overall
daily food intake to no more than 1,550
calories per day while adding a wider variety
of foods, which will include whole grains,
fruits, and low-fat dairy goods such as yogurt
and cheese. The lean and green diet also
provides additional tools to aid weight loss
and maintenance, which includes tips and
inspiration, community forums, weekly
support calls, and an app that allows you to set
meal reminders to track your food intake and
your activity level.*

*In short, the lean and green diet is designed to
help people lose weight and fat by reducing
calories and carbs through portion-controlled
meals and snacks. Its basis consists of
reduced-carbs programs that combine
processed, packaged calorie-counted foods*

with homemade meals that encourage weight loss. You can choose from several options; they all include products called "Fueling" as well as homemade meals, which follow the lean and green carb-fat ratio. The fueling comprises over 60 items low in carbs, but high in protein and probiotic cultures. These friendly bacteria can boost your gut health. These items include snack bars, cookies, shakes, puddings, cereals, soups, and pasta. All super-convenient and nutritious, while designed to help you feel satisfied.

13

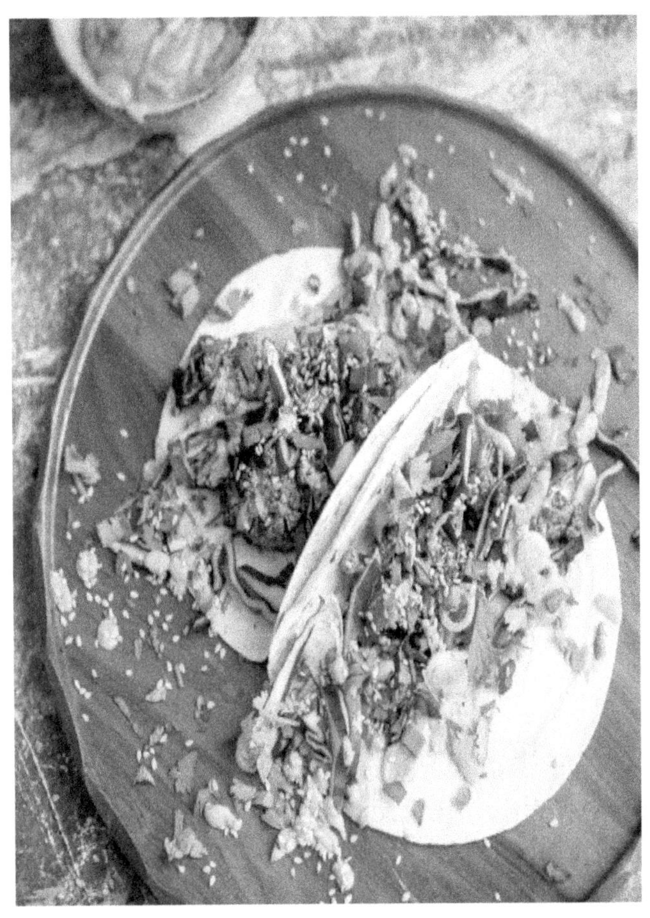

(Ready in a brief time frame, Serve 6, Difficulty: Normal) Nutrition per Serving: Calories: 335, Proteins: 13.8 g, Carbohydrates: 60.1 g, Fat: 4.3 g

Fixings:

- tablespoon of olive oil
- cloves of garlic, minced
- ½ red onion, minced
- ½ cup of red ring pepper, julienned
- ½ cup of julienned carrots
- ½ cup of dry red wine
- 1 cup of rehydrated porcini mushrooms
- 1 ½ cup of crushed tomatoes
- teaspoons of cut new basil
- 1 teaspoon of dried rosemary, crushed
- Salt and pepper, to taste

- 6 cups of tagliatelle

Bearings:

1. Over medium hotness, heat the oil in a gigantic skillet. Add garlic and onions and cook for 4 minutes, then, add the red toll pepper and carrots and cook for 4 extra minutes. Add the red wine, increase the hotness, cook for 1 second, lessen the hotness to medium-low, cook for 3 minutes after adding garlic.

2. Add the tomatoes, basil, and rosemary, season to taste with salt and pepper.

3. Stew for 10 minutes, then, serve over scorched noodles with sauce.

(Ready in a brief time frame, Serve 4, Difficulty: Normal) Nutrition per Serving: Calories: 287, Proteins: 15.1 g, Carbohydrates: 76.8 g, Fat: 13.2 g, Cholesterol: 0 mg, Sodium: 1248.8 mg.

Fixings:

o tablespoon olive oil

o ¼ cup finely divided onion

o 1(15.5 ounces) can dim saw peas, exhausted

o ½ cup vegetable stock

o 1 new jalapeno pepper, separated

o 1 clove of garlic, minced

o 1 tablespoon of new lime juice

o Salt and pepper, to taste

o 4(12 inches) flour tortillas

Headings:

1. Heat the olive oil over medium hotness in a medium skillet and cook the onion until it is sensitive.

2. Join the dim took a gander at peas, vegetable save, jalapeno, lime juice, and garlic cloves Season to taste with salt and pepper, and continue to cook until hot.

3. Encase the mix by the tortillas to serve.

(Arranged without further ado, Serve 2, Difficulty: Easy) Nutrition per Serving: Calories: 129, Proteins: 18 g, Carbohydrates: 111.9 g, Fat: 10.6 g, Cholesterol: 0 mg, Sodium: 314.5 mg.

Fixings:

o 2 whole star anise units

o Salt, to taste

o 3 cloves of garlic, stripped and divided

o ½ red ringer pepper, divided

o 2 dried hot red peppers, diced

o ½ teaspoon of ground dim pepper

o 4 colossal new mushrooms, separated

o tablespoon of lemon juice

o ¼ cup of separated dates

o 1 teaspoon of ground cinnamon

o 1 cup of uncooked couscous

o 1 ½ cups of vegetable stock

Bearings:

1. Heat the oil over low hotness in a medium pot, and sauté the onion until it is fragile. Using the anise cases and salt to get ready. Blend the garlic, red ringer pepper, lively dried red peppers, and dim pepper.

2. Blend in the vegetable mix in with the mushrooms and lemon juice. Incorporate the dates and cinnamon, and cook for around 10 minutes over low hotness.

3. In a medium skillet, position the couscous and cover with vegetable stock. Heat it with the end result of bubbling. Reduce hotness to low levels. Cover and air pocket until the clamminess has been exhausted, 3-5 minutes.

4. With a fork, mix in the vegetables and eat. Pad couscous.

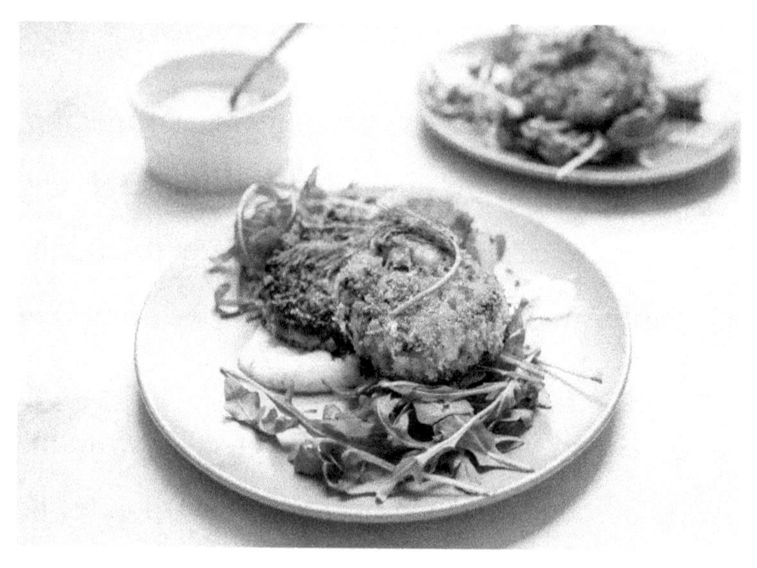

(Ready in an hour, Serve 6, Difficulty: Normal) Nutrition per Serving: Calories: 149, Proteins: 4.2 g, Carbohydrates: 23.5 g, Fat: 4.9 g, Cholesterol: 0 mg, Sodium: 650.5 mg.

Fixings:

o 680 g of red potatoes, cut into knots

o 2 tablespoons virgin olive oil

o 8 cloves of garlic, gently cut

o 4 teaspoons of dried rosemary

o 4 teaspoons of dried thyme

o 2 teaspoons of authentic salt

o bunch of new asparagus, oversaw and cut into 1-inch pieces

o Ground dim pepper to taste

Bearings:

1. 425 degrees Fahrenheit when preheating.

2. In an enormous baking dish, toss the red potatoes with ½ the olive oil, garlic, rosemary, thyme, and ½ the veritable salt. Cover with aluminum foil.

3. Get ready 20 minutes in the preheated oven. Mix in the asparagus, remaining olive oil, and remaining salt. Cook when covered for 15 minutes, or until the potatoes are fragile. Increase oven temperature to 450 degrees Fahrenheit (232 degrees Celsius).

4. Kill foil, and continue to cook 5-10 minutes, until potatoes are gently sautéed. Season with pepper to serve.

Veggie lover Holiday Roast with Mashed Vegetables

(Ready in a brief time frame, Serve 4-6, Difficulty: Easy) Nutrition per Serving: Calories: 246, Proteins: 19 g, Carbohydrates: 22 g, Fat: 9 g, Fiber: 3g.

Fixings:

o 1, 1 lb. (thawed out) veggie sweetheart stuffed cook

o 2 cups diced potato

o 2 cups diced carrots

o cup diced yellow onion

o ¾-1 cup of veggie stock

o 4 minced garlic cloves

o 1 tablespoon almond milk

o 1 teaspoon olive oil

o Salt and pepper to taste

Rules:

1. In your strain cooker, heat the oil.

2. Cook the garlic and onion for brief when it is hot.

3. Add the vegetables, salt, and potatoes and join.

4. On top of the vegetables, put the feast on top and flood the stock.

5. Cover the top and seal it

6. Select 'manual' and cook for 8 minutes at low strain or around 6 minutes at high pressure.

7. Hit 'drop' and quick conveyance when the time is up.

8. Let the dinner out.

9. For the vegetables, add almond milk and pepper and smash to your ideal consistency.

10. Serve.

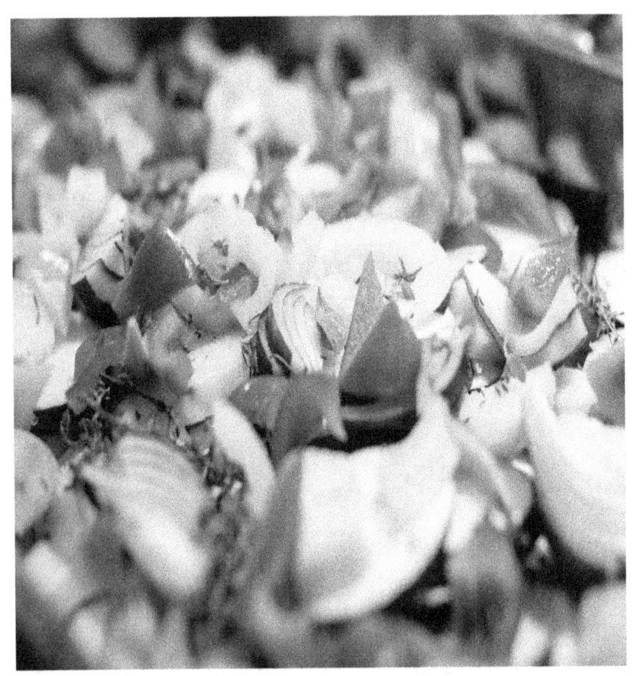

(Ready in a brief time frame, Serve 4, Difficulty: Easy) Nutrition per Serving: Calories: 328, Proteins: 18 g, Carbohydrates: 51.9 g, Fat: 8.3 g, Cholesterol: .7 mg, Sodium: 633 mg.

Fixings:

o cup of red lentils

o ¼ cup of tomato puree

o ½ (8 ounces) compartment of plain yogurt

o 1 teaspoon of garam masala

o ½ teaspoon of ground dried turmeric

o ½ teaspoon of ground cumin

o ½ teaspoon of Ancho chile powder

o tablespoons of vegetable oil

o 1 onion, separated

o cloves of garlic, separated

o 1(1 inch) piece new ginger root, ground

o cups of roughly squeezed new spinach, coarsely divided

o 2 tomatoes, separated

o sprigs of new cilantro, separated

o 1(15.5 ounces) container of mixed beans, washed and drained.

Rules:

1. Flush the lentils and put adequate water in a container to cover them. Heat it with the eventual result of bubbling. Cut down the hotness, cover the pot and air pocket for 20 minutes over low hotness, channel.

2. Blend the tomato puree and yogurt together in a dish. Season with garam masala, turmeric, stew powder, and cumin. Dispose of before smooth.

3. Heat oil over low hotness in a dish. Add the onion, garlic, and ginger, then, stew until the onion starts to brown. Blend in the spinach, then, stew until withered and faint green. Blend

in the yogurt mix one small step at a time.
Then, the tomatoes and cilantro are solidified.
4. Blend in the mix of lentils and mixed beans
once even. Heat through, 5 minutes, generally.

(Ready in 1 hour and 35 minutes, Serve 1, Difficulty: Hard) Nutrition per Serving: Calories: 218, Proteins: 6.2 g, Carbohydrates: 29.8 g, Fat: 5.2 g, Cholesterol: 0 mg, Sodium: 147.1 mg.

Fixings:

o 2 cups of vegetable stock, secluded

o teaspoon of yeast separate spread, (as Marmite®/Vegemite®)

o ½ cup dry lentils

o ¼ cup of pearl grain

o 1 tremendous carrot, diced

o ½ onion, finely hacked

o ½ cup of walnuts, coarsely hacked

o potatoes, severed

o 1 teaspoon of for the most part valuable flour

o ½ teaspoon of water

o Salt and pepper, to taste

Bearings:

1. 350 degrees Fahrenheit (176 degrees Celsius) when preheating on the oven.

2. Solidify, ¼ cups of stock, yeast concentrate, lentils, and grain in a tremendous container over medium-low hotness. For 30 minutes, bubble.

3. Meanwhile, mix the overabundance 3⁄4 cup stock, carrot, onion, and walnuts in a medium pot and cook until fragile, around 15 minutes.

4. Meanwhile, put it to a flood with a significant pot of salted water. Add the potatoes and cook for around 15 minutes, until fragile yet solid. Squash and wash.

5. Mix the flour and water, blend in the carrot mix and air pocket until thickened. Join a mix of carrots with a blend of lentils and season with salt and pepper. Void the blend into a

bowl of 2 quarts of feast. Spoon burned potatoes over a blend of lentils.

6. Plan in a preheated oven for around 30 minutes, until finely carmelized on top.

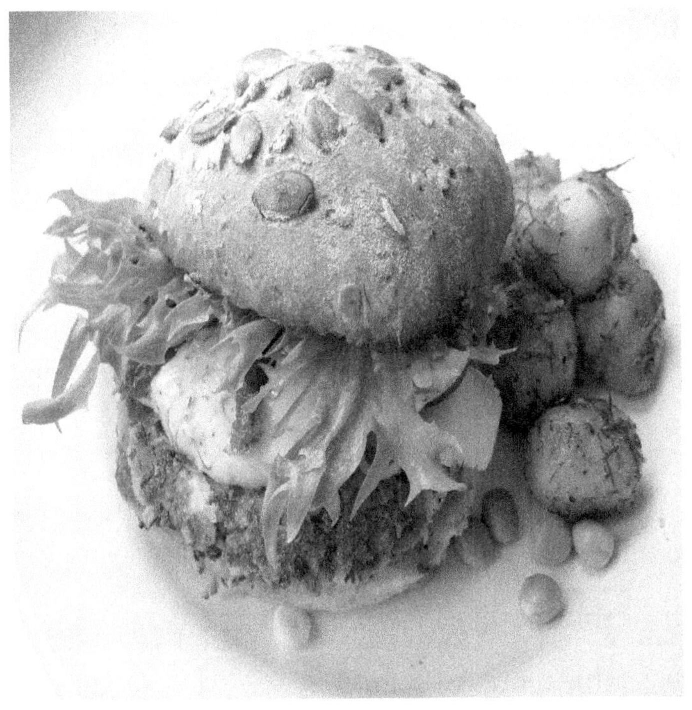

(Arranged instantly, Serve 4, Difficulty: Normal) Nutrition per Serving: Calories: 198, Proteins: 11.2 g, Carbohydrates: 33.1 g, Fat: 3 g, Cholesterol: 46.5 mg, Sodium: 607.3 mg.

Fixings:

o 1(16 ounces) holder of dim beans, exhausted and washed

o ½ green ring pepper, cut into 2-inch pieces

o ½ onion, cut into wedges

o 3 cloves of garlic, stripped

o egg

o 1 tablespoon of stew powder

o 1 tablespoon of cumin

o 1 teaspoon of Thai stew sauce or hot sauce

o ½ cup bread pieces

Bearings:

1. While grilling, preheat a high-heat grill and carefully oil a sheet of aluminum foil. Preheat the oven before baking, and carefully oil your baking sheet.

2. Pulverize the dim beans with a fork in a medium bowl until they are thick and pale.

3. Cut the toll pepper, onion, and garlic gently in a food processor. Blend in the squashed beans, then.

4. Blend the egg, stew powder, and stew sauce together in a little cup.

5. Blend in the squashed beans with the egg mix. Until the paste is sodden and remains together, incorporate bread scraps. Break the blend into 4-patties.

6. *While grilling, put the patties on the foil and grill on either side for around 8 minutes. While baking, put the patties on the baking sheet and plan on each side for around 10 minutes*

Red Lentil Curry

(Prepared shortly, Serve 8, Difficulty: Normal)

Nutrition per Serving: Calories: 219, Proteins: 12.1 g, Carbohydrates: 32.5 g, Fat: 2.6 g, Cholesterol: 0 mg, Sodium: 571.9 mg.

Ingredients:

o   *2 cups of red lentils*

o   *large onion, diced*

o   *1 tablespoon of vegetable oil*

o   *tablespoons of curry glue*

o   *1 tablespoon of curry powder*

o   *1 teaspoon of ground turmeric*

o   *1 teaspoon of ground cumin*

o   *1 teaspoon of stew powder*

o   *1 teaspoon of salt*

o   *1 teaspoon white sugar*

o   *1 teaspoon of minced garlic*

o   *1 teaspoon of minced new ginger*

o   *1(14.25 ounces) container of tomato puree.*

Directions:

1. Wash the lentils until the water runs clean in chilly water. Place the lentils in a pot with sufficient water to cover, heat to the point of boiling, put a cover on the pot, diminish hotness to medium-low, and stew, adding water for 15-20 minutes during cooking, as expected, until delicate. Channel.

2. Heat the vegetable oil over medium hotness in a huge skillet, cook and mix the onions in the hot oil until they are caramelized around 20 minutes.

3. In a major bowl, consolidate the curry glue, curry powder, turmeric, stew powder, cinnamon, sugar, garlic, and ginger. Mix in the onions. Help the fire to high and stew for 1-2 minutes, mixing constantly, until fragrant.

4. Eliminate from the hotness, mix in the tomato puree and mix in the lentils.

(Prepared quickly, Serve 10, Difficulty: Easy)

Nutrition per Serving: Calories: 140, Proteins: 6.3 g, Carbohydrates: 27.1 g, Fat: 0.9 g, Cholesterol: 0 mg, Sodium: 354.4 mg.

Ingredients:

o   *teaspoon of olive oil*

o   *1 onion, slashed*

o   *cloves of garlic, minced*

o   *¾ cup of uncooked white rice*

o   *1 ½ cups of low Sodium:, low-fat vegetable stock*

o   *1 teaspoon of ground cumin*

o	¼ teaspoon of cayenne pepper

o	3 ½ cups of canned dark beans, depleted

Directions:

1. Heat the oil in a stockpot over medium-high hotness. Add the garlic and onion and cook for 4 minutes. For 2 minutes, add the rice and sauté.

2. Cook for 20 minutes, add the vegetable stock, heat to the point of boiling, cover, and lower the tension. Add the dark beans and preparing.

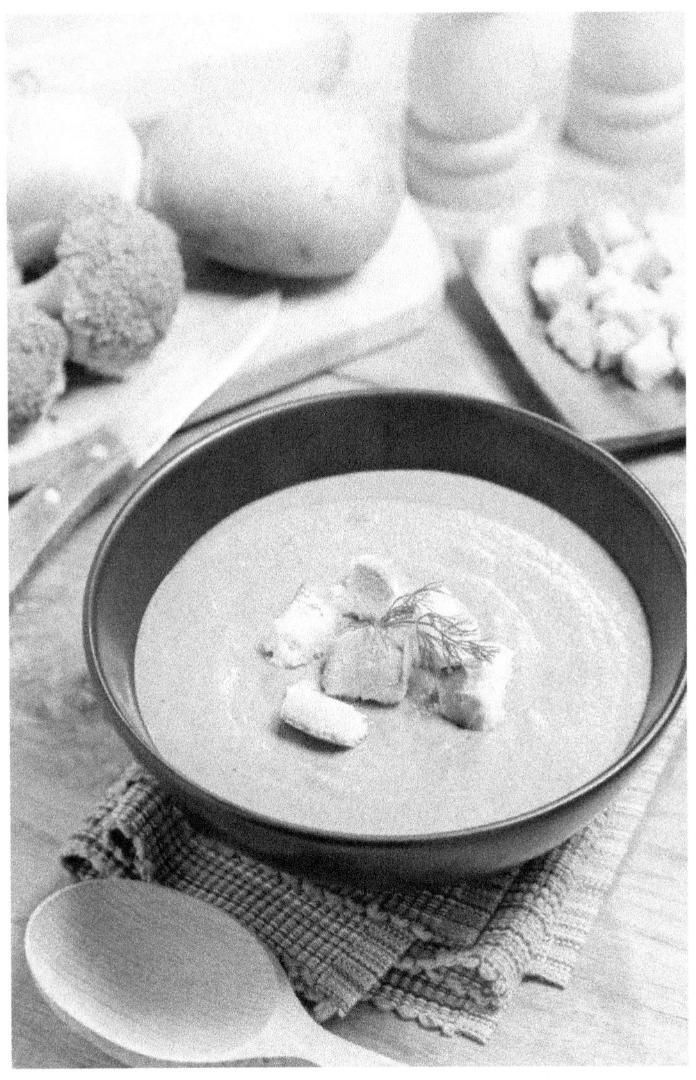

(Prepared in 1 hour and 10 minutes, Serve 8, Difficulty: Normal) Nutrition per Serving: Calories: 112, Protein: 18.7 g, Carbohydrates: 17.8 g, Fat: 11.2 g, Cholesterol: 51.7 mg, Sodium: 950.4 mg.

Ingredients:

- *680 g of ground hamburger*

o *1 medium onion, finely slashed*

- *3(14.5 ounces) jars of hamburger consommé*

- *1(28 ounces) jar of diced tomatoes*

- *2 cups of water*

- *1(10.75 ounces) jar of consolidated tomato soup*

- *4 carrots, finely slashed*

- *3 stems of celery, finely slashed*

- *4 tablespoons of pearl grain*

- *½ teaspoon of dried thyme*

- *narrows leaf*

Guidelines:

Rules:

1. Switch on a multi-valuable strain cooker and select the cook mode (like Instant Pot®). Cook and blend until carmelized, 5-10 minutes, with the meat and onion. Pour the burger, onions, water, and tomato soup into the mix. Add some celery, onions, grain, thyme, and river leaf.

2. Cover the top and lock it. Pick "Part Soup," set the clock to 30 minutes. Grant strain to labor for 10-15 minutes.

3. The conveyance pressure is around 10 minutes including the ordinary conveyance procedure as instructed by the maker.

(Prepared in a short time, Serve 4, Difficulty: Normal) Nutrition per Serving: Calories: 138, Protein: 15.7 g, Carbohydrates: 25.9 g, Fat: 24.7 g, Cholesterol: 74.9 mg, Sodium: 367.6 mg.

Ingredients:

- *¾ cup of water*

o *1 cup of cleaved cauliflower*

- *1 cup of cubed potatoes*

- *½ cup of finely cleaved celery*

- *½ cup of diced carrots*

- *¼ cup of cleaved onion*

- *¼ cup of margarine*

- *¼ cup of universally handy flour*

o *3 cups of milk*

- *Salt and pepper, to taste*

o *4 ounces of destroyed cheddar*

Headings:

1. Unite the water, cauliflower, carrots, potatoes, celery, and onion in a tremendous container. It should be risen for 5-10 minutes, or until sensitive. Just set aside.

2. Over medium pressure, melt the margarine in an alternate container. Add the flour, then, stew for 2 minutes.

3. Kill from the hotness, and blend in the milk ceaselessly. Return to the hotness and stew until the mix thickens. With the cooking liquid, blend in the vegetables and season with salt

and pepper. Kill from the hotness and rush in
the cheddar until mellowed.

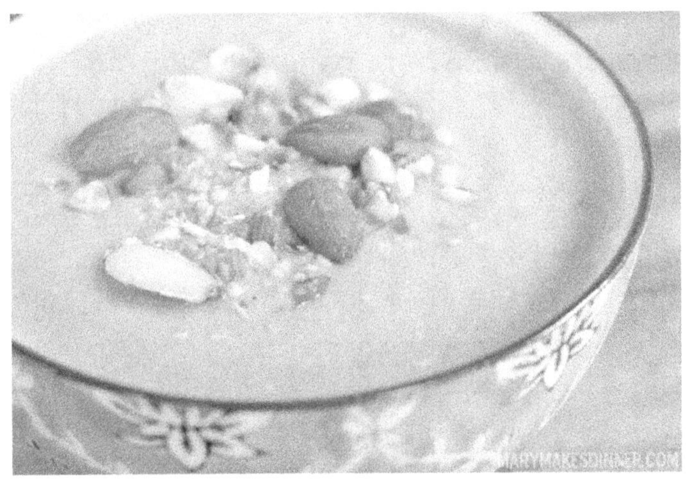

Culinary specialist John's Butternut Bisque

(Prepared shortly, Serve 6, Difficulty: Normal) Nutrition per Serving: Calories: 213, Protein: 3.2 g, Carbohydrates: 27.1 g, Fat: 13.7 g, Cholesterol 45.8 mg, Sodium: 1058.9 mg.

Ingredients:

- *3 tablespoons of spread*

o *1 huge onion, diced*

- *1 teaspoon of legitimate salt, in addition to additional to taste, partitioned*

- *1(907 g) butternut squash*

o *2 tablespoons of tomato glue*

o   *quart of chicken stock*

o   *1 touch of cayenne pepper*

o   *tablespoons of maple syrup, or to taste*

o   *½ cup of weighty cream or crème fraiche*

o   *Pomegranate seeds*

o   *For Garnish:*

o   *Some weighty cream or crème fraiche*

o   *Chopped new chives.*

Bearings:

1. Over medium-low pressure, break up spread in a pot. Put in the onions and a tremendous dash of salt. Cook and blend until the onions, around 10-15 minutes, have mellowed at this point not taken on any tone.

2. Eliminate the squash closes. Carefully cut the squash the long way in ½ and dispense with

the seeds. Using a potato peeler, strip the squash. Cut into bumps.

3. Raise the hotness to medium-high underneath the pot. In the tomato stick, blend, stew, and blend until the mix starts to caramelize and brown for around 2 minutes. Add the potato, 1 teaspoon of salt, chicken stock, and cayenne pepper. Hotness with the end result of bubbling, reduce hotness to medium-low, and stew, 15-25 minutes, until the squash is incredibly fragile. Decrease hotness to low levels. Blend until truly smooth with a submersion blender. Add the cream and maple syrup and if important, add more salt.

4. Spoon into bowls for serving. decorate with a cream spin and a disseminating of pomegranate seeds and chives.

Yam, Carrot, Apple, and Red Lentil Soup

(Prepared in 1 hour and 10 minutes, Serve 6, Difficulty: Normal) Nutrition per Serving: Calories: 232, Protein: 9 g, Carbohydrates: 52.9 g, Fat: 9 g, Cholesterol: 21.6 mg, Sodium: 876.3 mg.

Ingredients:

o *¼ cup of margarine*

o *2 enormous yams, stripped and slashed*

o *3 enormous carrots, stripped and slashed*

o *apple, stripped, cored, and slashed*

o *1 onion, slashed*

o *½ cup of red lentils*

o   ½ teaspoon of minced new ginger

o   ½ teaspoon of ground dark pepper

o   1 teaspoon of salt

o   ½ teaspoon of ground cumin

o   ½ teaspoon of bean stew powder

o   ½ teaspoon of paprika

o   4 cups of vegetable stock

o   Plain yogurt

Bearings:

1. Break down the spread over medium-high hotness in a significant profound lined pot. In the pot, unite the divided sweet potatoes, carrots, apple, and onion. Blend and cook the apples and vegetables for around 10 minutes before the onions are clear.

2. In a pot with the apple and vegetable mix, blend the lentils, ginger, ground dim pepper,

cinnamon, stew powder, paprika, and vegetable stock. Heat the soup with the eventual result of bubbling over high hotness, then, decline the hotness to medium-low, cover and stew for around 30 minutes until the lentils and vegetables are sensitive.

3. Void the soup into a blender, working in packs, filling the pitcher something like for the most part full. With an imploded kitchen towel, hold the blender's cover down and start the blender circumspectly, using several short pulses to move the soup before giving it to puree. Purée until smooth and fill a perfect pot in bunches. Then again, straightforwardly in the cooking pot, you ought to use a stick blender to puree the stock.

4. Place the pureed soup back in the cooking pot. Bring back over medium-high hotness, around 10 minutes, to a stew. To thin the soup to your ideal consistency, add water contingent

upon the circumstance. For embellish, present with yogurt.

5. Instead of yogurt as an improvement, this soup is in like manner particularly presented with broke down feta cheddar.

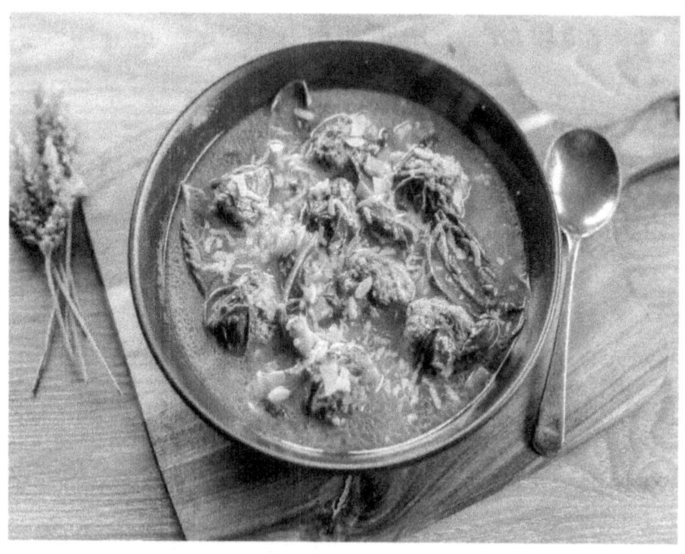

(Prepared quickly, Serve 6, Difficulty: Easy) Nutrition per Serving: Calories: 159, Protein: 11.5 g, Carbohydrates: 15.4 g, Fat: 5.6 g, Cholesterol:55.3 mg, Sodium: 98.6 mg.

Ingredients:

o   *226 g of extra-lean ground meat*

o   *egg, daintily beaten*

o   *tablespoons   of   Italian-prepared breadcrumbs*

o   *1 tablespoon of ground parmesan cheddar*

o   *tablespoons of destroyed new basil leaves*

o	*1 tablespoon of hacked Italian level leaf parsley (Optional)*

o	*2 green onions, cut (Optional)*

o	*5 ¾ cups of chicken stock*

o	*2 cups of finely cut escarole (spinach might be subbed)*

o	*1 lemon, zested*

o	*½ cup of orzo (rice-formed pasta), uncooked*

For Topping:

o	*Grated parmesan cheddar*

Rules:

1. The meat, egg, parsley, bread pieces, cheddar, basil, and green onions are mixed to shape 3/4-inch balls.

2. Over high hotness, void the stock into an enormous pot. Drop into meatballs while

foaming. Blend in escarole, orzo, and lemon punch. Return to an air pocket and decline to medium hotness. Cook for 10 minutes on a languid air pocket or until the orzo is fragile, blending a large part of the time. Present with cheddar.

Veggie lover Kale Soup

(Prepared shortly, Serve 8, Difficulty: Normal)

Nutrition per Serving: Calories: 277, Protein: 9.6 g, Carbohydrates: 50.9 g, Fat: 4.5 g, Cholesterol: 0 mg, Sodium: 372.2 mg.

Ingredients:

o	2 tablespoons of olive oil

o	yellow onion, hacked

o	tablespoons of hacked garlic

o	1 pack of kale, stems eliminated and leaves cleaved

o	8 cups of water

o	6 3D shapes of vegetable bouillon (like Knorr®)

o	1(15 ounces) jar of diced tomatoes

o   *6 white potatoes, stripped and cubed*

o   *2(15 ounces) jars of cannellini beans (depleted whenever wanted)*

o   *1 tablespoon of Italian flavoring*

o   *tablespoons of dried parsley*

o   *Salt and pepper, to taste*

Headings:

1. In an immense soup pot, heat the olive oil and cook the onion and garlic until sensitive. Blend in the kale and cook for around 2 minutes, until withered. Blend in the water, stir up the water

2. Tomatoes, potatoes, beans, vegetable bouillon, Italian seasoning, and parsley. Stew the soup for 25 minutes on medium hotness or until the potatoes are totally cooked. To taste, season with salt and pepper.

(Prepared quickly, Serve 6, Difficulty: Normal)

Nutrition per Serving: Calories: 130, Protein: 16.4 g, Carbohydrates: 16.8 g, Fat: 23.1 g, Cholesterol: 36.8 mg, Sodium: 662.9 mg.

Ingredients:

o   *2 tablespoons of red curry glue*

o   *red chime pepper, daintily cut*

o   *1 little onion, hacked*

o   *1(14 ounces) jar of coconut milk*

o   *1 tablespoon of fish sauce*

o   *cups of natively constructed chicken stock*

o   *cups of destroyed cooked chicken*

o   *1 ½ cups of cooked basmati rice*

o   *tablespoons of slashed new cilantro*

Guidelines:

Rules:

1. Cook the curry stick over medium-high hotness in a colossal, profound dish until the oils are set to convey, 1-2 minutes. Add the red pepper and onion and cook for around 5 minutes, blending, until sensitive. Blend in coconut milk until mixed well. Add the fish sauce, and afterward, by then, the stock of chicken.

2. Cut down the hotness and stew for 15 minutes. Add cooked rice and chicken. Blend over heat until totally warmed. Only preceding serving, add severed cilantro.

(Prepared in 1 hour and 20 minutes, Serve 8, Difficulty: Hard) Nutrition per Serving: Calories: 266, Protein: 5.1 g, Carbohydrates: 33.8 g, Fat: 14.5 g, Cholesterol: 42.2 mg, Sodium: 139.3 mg.

Ingredients:

o	butternut squash, split and cultivated

o	1 oak seed squash, split and cultivated

o	tablespoons of margarine

o	¼ cup of slashed sweet onion

o	1 quart of chicken stock

o	1 cup of pressed earthy colored sugar

o   1(8 ounces) bundle of cream cheddar, relaxed

o   ½ teaspoon of ground dark pepper

o   ½ teaspoon of ground cinnamon to taste

o   Fresh parsley, for embellish

Directions:

1. Preheat the stove to 350 degrees Fahrenheit (176 degrees Celsius). Place the side-cut squash parts in a baking dish. Heat until delicate or 45 minutes. Eliminate from the hotness and marginally cool. Scoop the skins with the mash and dispose of.

2. Liquefy the margarine over medium hotness in a skillet, and sauté the onion until it is delicate.

3. Blend the squash mash, onion, cream cheddar, stock, earthy colored sugar, pepper, and cinnamon in a blender or food processor until smooth. This can be completed in a few clumps.

4. Move the soup over medium hotness to a pot and cook, once in a while blending, until completely warmed. Decorate with parsley and warm to serve.

(Prepared quickly, Serve 6, Difficulty: Normal)

Nutrition per Serving: Calories: 14, Protein: 7 g, Carbohydrates: 16.2 g, Fat: 7 g, Cholesterol: 18.9 mg, Sodium: 573.1 mg.

Ingredients:

o   *2 tablespoons of unsalted margarine*

o   *2 cups of slashed onions*

o   *680 g of new mushrooms, thickly cut*

o   *4 ½ teaspoons of slashed new dill*

o   *tablespoon of Hungarian sweet paprika*

o   *1 tablespoon of soy sauce*

o   *cups of low-sodium chicken stock*

o   1 cup of skim milk

o   tablespoons of universally handy flour

o   ½ ready tomato

o   ½ Hungarian wax pepper

o   teaspoon of salt

o   Ground dark pepper, to taste

o   ½ cup of light harsh cream.

Guidelines:

1. In a huge pot over medium hotness, dissolve the margarine. In the spread, cook and mix the onions until fragrant, around 5 minutes. Add the mushrooms and keep on cooking for around 5 additional minutes until the mushrooms are delicate. Blend the mushroom combination in with the dill, paprika, soy

sauce, and chicken stock, lessen the hotness to low, cover and stew for 15 minutes.

2. In a little bowl, whisk the milk and the flour together. In the soup, mix the combination. Add the Hungarian wax and tomato pepper. Return the cover to the pot and stew, at times blending, for an additional 15 minutes. With salt and pepper, season.

3. In the soup, join the harsh cream and proceed to cook and mix until the soup has thickened, 5-10 additional minutes. Eliminate the pepper and tomato from the Hungarian wax and dispose of them prior to serving the soup.

(Prepared in 1 hour and 5 minutes, Serve 10, Difficulty: Normal) Nutrition per Serving: Calories: 257, Protein: 10.1 g, Carbohydrates: 24.4 g, Fat: 13.8 g, Cholesterol: 31 mg, Sodium: 626.3 mg.

Ingredients:

- *1(16 ounces) bundle of pork frankfurter*

- *3 medium beets, stripped and destroyed*

- *3 carrots, stripped and destroyed*

- *3 medium baking potatoes, stripped and cubed*

o *tablespoon of vegetable oil*

- *1 medium onion, slashed*

- *1(6 ounces) jar of tomato glue*

- *¾ cup of water*

- *½ medium head cabbage, cored and destroyed*

- *1(8 ounces) jar of diced tomatoes, depleted*

o *cloves of garlic, minced*

- *Salt and pepper, to taste*

- *1 teaspoon of white sugar, or to taste*

For Topping:

- *½ cup of sharp cream*

For Garnish:

- *1 tablespoon of slashed new parsley*

Guidelines:

1. Disintegrate (if utilizing the frankfurter over medium-high hotness into a skillet. Cook and mix until it isn't pink any longer. Eliminate and save from the hotness.

2. Fill an enormous pot with water mostly (around 2 quarts) and heat it to the point of boiling. Mix in the wiener, then, at that point, cover the pot. Get back to a bubble. Add the beets, and cook until their shading is no more. Add the carrots and potatoes, and cook for around 15 minutes, until delicate. Add the cabbage, the diced tomatoes, and the can.

3. Over medium hotness, heat the oil in a skillet. Add the onion, then, at that point, cook until it's delicate. Join the tomato glue and water until very much blended. To the pot, move. To the soup, add the crude garlic, cover, and turn the hotness off. Allow them to stand

for 5 minutes. Taste, and then, at that point, season with salt, sugar, and pepper.

4. Scoop it into serving bowls and whenever wanted, decorate it with harsh cream and new parsley.

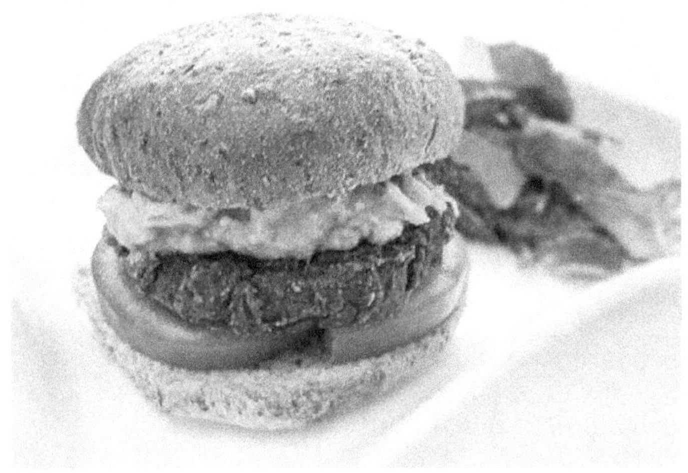

(Arranged instantly, Serve 4, Difficulty: Normal) Nutrition per Serving: Calories: 198, Proteins: 11.2 g, Carbohydrates: 33.1 g, Fat: 3 g, Cholesterol: 46.5 mg, Sodium: 607.3 mg.

Fixings:

o 1(16 ounces) holder of dim beans, exhausted and washed

o ½ green ring pepper, cut into 2-inch pieces

o ½ onion, cut into wedges

o 3 cloves of garlic, stripped

o egg

o 1 tablespoon of stew powder

o 1 tablespoon of cumin

o 1 teaspoon of Thai stew sauce or hot sauce

o ½ cup bread pieces

Bearings:

1. While grilling, preheat a high-heat grill and carefully oil a sheet of aluminum foil. Preheat the oven before baking, and carefully oil your baking sheet.

2. Pulverize the dim beans with a fork in a medium bowl until they are thick and pale.

3. Cut the toll pepper, onion, and garlic gently in a food processor. Blend in the squashed beans, then.

4. Blend the egg, stew powder, and stew sauce together in a little cup.

5. Blend in the squashed beans with the egg mix. Until the paste is sodden and remains together, incorporate bread scraps. Break the blend into 4-patties.

6. While grilling, put the patties on the foil and grill on either side for around 8 minutes. While baking, put the patties on the baking sheet and plan on each side for around 10 minutes

(Prepared shortly, Serve 8, Difficulty: Normal)

Nutrition per Serving: Calories: 219, Proteins: 12.1 g, Carbohydrates: 32.5 g, Fat: 2.6 g, Cholesterol: 0 mg, Sodium: 571.9 mg.

Ingredients:

o   *2 cups of red lentils*

o   *large onion, diced*

o   *1 tablespoon of vegetable oil*

o   *tablespoons of curry glue*

o   *1 tablespoon of curry powder*

o   *1 teaspoon of ground turmeric*

o   *1 teaspoon of ground cumin*

o   *1 teaspoon of stew powder*

o   *1 teaspoon of salt*

o   *1 teaspoon white sugar*

o   *1 teaspoon of minced garlic*

o   *1 teaspoon of minced new ginger*

o   *1(14.25 ounces) container of tomato puree.*

Directions:

1. Wash the lentils until the water runs clean in chilly water. Place the lentils in a pot with sufficient water to cover, heat to the point of boiling, put a cover on the pot, diminish hotness to medium-low, and stew, adding water for 15-20 minutes during cooking, as expected, until delicate. Channel.

2. Heat the vegetable oil over medium hotness in a huge skillet, cook and mix the onions in the hot oil until they are caramelized around 20 minutes.

3. In a major bowl, consolidate the curry glue, curry powder, turmeric, stew powder, cinnamon, sugar, garlic, and ginger. Mix in the onions. Help the fire to high and stew for 1-2 minutes, mixing constantly, until fragrant.

4. Eliminate from the hotness, mix in the tomato puree and mix in the lentils.

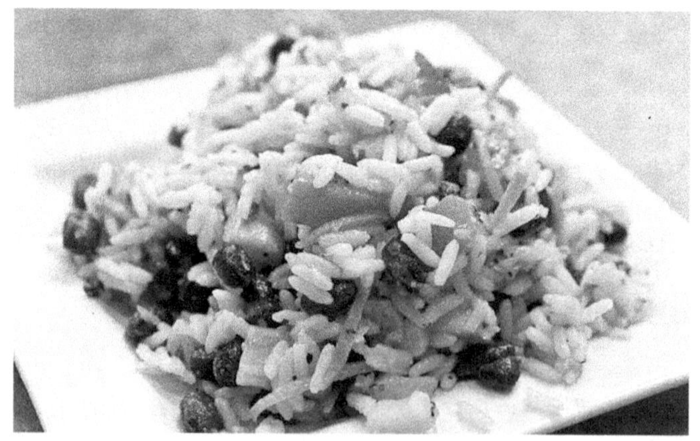

(Prepared quickly, Serve 10, Difficulty: Easy) Nutrition per Serving: Calories: 140, Proteins: 6.3 g, Carbohydrates: 27.1 g, Fat: 0.9 g, Cholesterol: 0 mg, Sodium: 354.4 mg.

Ingredients:

o   *teaspoon of olive oil*

o   *1 onion, slashed*

o   *cloves of garlic, minced*

o   *¾ cup of uncooked white rice*

o   *1 ½ cups of low Sodium, low-fat vegetable stock*

o   *1 teaspoon of ground cumin*

o   ¼ teaspoon of cayenne pepper

o   3 ½ cups of canned dark beans, depleted

Directions:

1. Heat the oil in a stockpot over medium-high hotness. Add the garlic and onion and cook for 4 minutes. For 2 minutes, add the rice and sauté.

2. Cook for 20 minutes, add the vegetable stock, heat to the point of boiling, cover, and lower the tension. Add the dark beans and preparing.

21 Day Meal Plan (5 & 1)

Day	5 Fueling Hacks (Breakfast & Lunch)	1 Lean & Green Meal (Dinner)
1	Virginia's Tuna Salad Green Lentils and Rice Assyrian Style Banana Pancakes Slow Cooked Corned Beef for Sandwiches Basic Italian Bean Soup	Smoky Vegan Black Bean Soup
2	Cardamom and Peach Quinoa Porridge Kale, Tomato and Poached Egg on Toast	Salmon with Grilled Eggplant and Chickpea Croutons

3	Porridge with Blueberry Compote Zesty Grilled Cheese Sandwich Well known in Italian Recipes	
	Eggy Spelt Bread with Orange Cheese and Raspberries Rich Mustard Mushrooms on Toast with A Glass of Juice Ham, Mushroom and Spinach Frittata Slow Cooker Italian Beef Sandwiches Slow Cooker Spicy Black-Eyed Peas	Mediterranean Chicken Bowls

4	Cranberry and Raspberry Smoothie Asparagus Soldiers with a Soft-Boiled Egg Honey Nut Crunch Pears Mother's Sushi Rice Barbecued Corn Salad	Sautéed Chicken with Lemony Roasted Broccoli
5	Honey Nut Crunch Pears Welsh Rarebit Muffins Hash Browns with Mustard and Smoked Salmon Measuring utencil's Vegetable Barley Soup Thin Taco Stuffed Peppers	Steak Salad with Charred Green Onions and Beets

6	*Eggy Spelt Bread with Orange Cheese and Raspberries* *Rich Mustard Mushrooms on Toast with A Glass of Juice* *Ham, Mushroom and Spinach Frittata* *Chicago-Inspired Italian Beef Sandwich* *Saturday Chicken Stock*	*Fish Poke Bowl Recipe*
7	*Cardamom and Peach Quinoa Porridge* *Kale, Tomato and Poached Egg on Toast* *Porridge with Blueberry Compote* *Smooth Sweet Tea*	*Provincial Smoky Glazed Chicken and Veggie Bake*

	Katie's Yogurt Veggie Salad	
8	Virginia's Tuna Salad Green Lentils and Rice Assyrian Style Banana Pancakes Slow Cooked Corned Beef for Sandwiches Basic Italian Bean Soup	Smoky Vegan Black Bean Soup
9	Cardamom and Peach Quinoa Porridge Kale, Tomato and Poached Egg on Toast Porridge with Blueberry Compote Zesty Grilled Cheese Sandwich	Salmon with Grilled Eggplant and Chickpea Croutons

	Well known in Italian Recipes	
10	*Eggy Spelt Bread with Orange Cheese and Raspberries* *Rich Mustard Mushrooms on Toast with A Glass of Juice* *Ham, Mushroom and Spinach Frittata* *Slow Cooker Italian Beef Sandwiches* *Slow Cooker Spicy Black-Eyed Peas*	*Mediterranean Chicken Bowls*
11	*Cranberry and Raspberry Smoothie* *Asparagus Soldiers with a Soft-Boiled Egg*	*Sautéed Chicken with Lemony Roasted Broccoli*

	Honey Nut Crunch Pears	
	Mother's Sushi Rice	
	Barbecued Corn Salad	
12	*Honey Nut Crunch Pears*	*Steak Salad with Charred Green Onions and Beets*
	Welsh Rarebit Muffins	
	Hash Browns with Mustard and Smoked Salmon	
	Measuring utencil's Vegetable Barley Soup	
	Thin Taco Stuffed Peppers	
13	*Eggy Spelt Bread with Orange Cheese and Raspberries*	*Fish Poke Bowl Recipe*

	Rich Mustard Mushrooms on Toast with A Glass of Juice *Ham, Mushroom and Spinach Frittata* *Chicago-Inspired Italian Beef Sandwich* *Saturday Chicken Stock*	
14	*Cardamom and Peach Quinoa Porridge* *Kale, Tomato and Poached Egg on Toast* *Porridge with Blueberry Compote* *Smooth Sweet Tea* *Katie's Yogurt Veggie Salad*	*Provincial Smoky Glazed Chicken and Veggie Bake*

15	Virginia's Tuna Salad Green Lentils and Rice Assyrian Style Banana Pancakes Slow Cooked Corned Beef for Sandwiches Basic Italian Bean Soup	Smoky Vegan Black Bean Soup
16	Cardamom and Peach Quinoa Porridge Kale, Tomato and Poached Egg on Toast Porridge with Blueberry Compote Zesty Grilled Cheese Sandwich Well known in Italian Recipes	Salmon with Grilled Eggplant and Chickpea Croutons

17	Eggy Spelt Bread with Orange Cheese and Raspberries Rich Mustard Mushrooms on Toast with A Glass of Juice Ham, Mushroom and Spinach Frittata Slow Cooker Italian Beef Sandwiches Slow Cooker Spicy Black-Eyed Peas	Mediterranean Chicken Bowls
18	Cranberry and Raspberry Smoothie Asparagus Soldiers with a Soft-Boiled Egg Honey Nut Crunch Pears	Sautéed Chicken with Lemony Roasted Broccoli

	Mother's Sushi Rice Barbecued Corn Salad	
19	Honey Nut Crunch Pears Welsh Rarebit Muffins Hash Browns with Mustard and Smoked Salmon Measuring utencil's Vegetable Barley Soup Thin Taco Stuffed Peppers	Steak Salad with Charred Green Onions and Beets
20	Eggy Spelt Bread with Orange Cheese and Raspberries Rich Mustard Mushrooms on Toast with A Glass of Juice	Fish Poke Bowl Recipe

	Ham, Mushroom and Spinach Frittata	
	Chicago-Inspired Italian Beef Sandwich	
	Saturday Chicken Stock	
21	*Cardamom and Peach Quinoa Porridge*	*Provincial Smoky Glazed Chicken and Veggie Bake*
	Kale, Tomato and Poached Egg on Toast	
	Porridge with Blueberry Compote	
	Smooth Sweet Tea	
	Katie's Yogurt Veggie Salad	

Day	4 Fueling Hacks	2 Lean & Green Meals	1 Snack
1	Virginia's Tuna Salad Banana Pancakes Slow Cooked Corned Beef for Sandwiches Basic Italian Bean Soup	Smoky Vegan Black Bean Soup Salmon with Grilled Eggplant and Chickpea Croutons	Porcini Mushroom Pasta
2	Cardamom and Peach Quinoa Porridge Porridge with Blueberry Compote Zesty Grilled Cheese Sandwich	Mediterranean Chicken Bowls Sautéed Chicken with Lemony Roasted Broccoli	Dark Eyed Peas and Tortillas

	Well known in Italian Recipes		
3	*Rich Mustard Mushrooms on Toast with A Glass of Juice* *Ham, Mushroom and Spinach Frittata* *Slow Cooker Italian Beef Sandwiches* *Slow Cooker Spicy Black-Eyed Peas*	*Steak Salad with Charred Green Onions and Beets* *Fish Poke Bowl Recipe*	*Hot Couscous with Dates*
4	*Asparagus Soldiers with a Soft-Boiled Egg* *Honey Nut Crunch Pears* *Mother's Sushi Rice*	*Provincial Smoky Glazed Chicken and Veggie Bake* *Smooth Corn Chowder*	*Broiler Roasted Red Potatoes and Asparagus*

	Barbecued Corn Salad		
5	*Honey Nut Crunch Pears* *Hash Browns with Mustard and Smoked Salmon* *Measuring utencil's Vegetable Barley Soup* *Thin Taco Stuffed Peppers*	*Moment Pot Chicken Soup* *Chicken Bolognese*	*Veggie lover Holiday Roast with Mashed Vegetables*
6	*Eggy Spelt Bread with Orange Cheese and Raspberries* *Rich Mustard Mushrooms on*	*Citrusy Shrimp-Stuffed Avocados* *Chicken Souvlaki Skewers*	*Spinach, Red Lentil, and Bean Curry*

	Toast with A Glass of Juice *Ham, Mushroom and Spinach Frittata* *Chicago-Inspired Italian Beef Sandwich*		
7	*Kale, Tomato and Poached Egg on Toast* *Porridge with Blueberry Compote* *Smooth Sweet Tea* *Katie's Yogurt* *Veggie Salad*	*Steak Chimichurri* *Caribbean Chicken and "Rice"*	*Vegan Shepherd's Pie*
8	*Virginia's Tuna Salad*	*Smoky Vegan Black Bean Soup*	*Porcini Mushroom Pasta*

	Banana Pancakes Slow Cooked Corned Beef for Sandwiches Basic Italian Bean Soup	Salmon with Grilled Eggplant and Chickpea Croutons	
9	Cardamom and Peach Quinoa Porridge Porridge with Blueberry Compote Zesty Grilled Cheese Sandwich Well known in Italian Recipes	Mediterranean Chicken Bowls Sautéed Chicken with Lemony Roasted Broccoli	Dark Eyed Peas and Tortillas
10	Rich Mustard Mushrooms on Toast with A Glass of Juice	Steak Salad with Charred Green Onions and Beets	Hot Couscous with Dates

	Ham, Mushroom and Spinach Frittata *Slow Cooker Italian Beef Sandwiches* *Slow Cooker Spicy Black-Eyed Peas*	*Fish Poke Bowl Recipe*	
11	*Asparagus Soldiers with a Soft-Boiled Egg* *Honey Nut Crunch Pears* *Mother's Sushi Rice* *Barbecued Corn Salad*	*Provincial Smoky Glazed Chicken and Veggie Bake* *Smooth Corn Chowder*	*Broiler Roasted Red Potatoes and Asparagus*
12	*Honey Nut Crunch Pears*	*Moment Pot Chicken Soup* *Chicken Bolognese*	*Veggie lover Holiday Roast with Mashed Vegetables*

	Hash Browns with Mustard and Smoked Salmon *Measuring utencil's Vegetable Barley Soup* *Thin Taco Stuffed Peppers*		
13	*Eggy Spelt Bread with Orange Cheese and Raspberries* *Rich Mustard Mushrooms on Toast with A Glass of Juice* *Ham, Mushroom and Spinach Frittata*	*Citrusy Shrimp-Stuffed Avocados* *Chicken Souvlaki Skewers*	*Spinach, Red Lentil, and Bean Curry*

	Chicago-Inspired Italian Beef Sandwich		
14	*Kale, Tomato and Poached Egg on Toast* *Porridge with Blueberry Compote* *Smooth Sweet Tea* *Katie's Yogurt Veggie Salad*	*Steak Chimichurri* *Caribbean Chicken and "Rice"*	*Vegan Shepherd's Pie*
15	*Virginia's Tuna Salad* *Banana Pancakes* *Slow Cooked Corned Beef for Sandwiches*	*Smoky Vegan Black Bean Soup* *Salmon with Grilled Eggplant and Chickpea Croutons*	*Porcini Mushroom Pasta*

	Basic Italian Bean Soup		
16	*Cardamom and Peach Quinoa Porridge* *Porridge with Blueberry Compote* *Zesty Grilled Cheese Sandwich* *Well known in Italian Recipes*	*Mediterranean Chicken Bowls* *Sautéed Chicken with Lemony Roasted Broccoli*	*Dark Eyed Peas and Tortillas*
17	*Rich Mustard Mushrooms on Toast with A Glass of Juice* *Ham, Mushroom and Spinach Frittata*	*Steak Salad with Charred Green Onions and Beets* *Fish Poke Bowl Recipe*	*Hot Couscous with Dates*

	Slow Cooker Italian Beef Sandwiches Slow Cooker Spicy Black-Eyed Peas		
18	Asparagus Soldiers with a Soft-Boiled Egg Honey Nut Crunch Pears Mother's Sushi Rice Barbecued Corn Salad	Provincial Smoky Glazed Chicken and Veggie Bake Smooth Corn Chowder	Broiler Roasted Red Potatoes and Asparagus
19	Honey Nut Crunch Pears Hash Browns with Mustard and Smoked Salmon	Moment Pot Chicken Soup Chicken Bolognese	Veggie lover Holiday Roast with Mashed Vegetables

	Measuring utencil's Vegetable Barley Soup *Thin Taco Stuffed Peppers*		
20	*Eggy Spelt Bread with Orange Cheese and Raspberries* *Rich Mustard Mushrooms on Toast with A Glass of Juice* *Ham, Mushroom and Spinach Frittata* *Chicago-Inspired Italian Beef Sandwich*	*Citrusy Shrimp-Stuffed Avocados* *Chicken Souvlaki Skewers*	*Spinach, Red Lentil, and Bean Curry*

| 21 | Kale, Tomato and Poached Egg on Toast

Porridge with Blueberry Compote

Smooth Sweet Tea

Katie's Yogurt

Veggie Salad | Steak Chimichurri

Caribbean Chicken and "Rice" | Vegan Shepherd's Pie |

The Plan 1 is the most commonly prescribed Lean and Green program because it is quite an effective one. The 5 and 1 recommends you to take six small meals in a day. The meals should be divided in such a way that there should be "5 Fuelings" meals and "1 lean and green" meal in a day. For this, you can select any of the fuelings and add to the diet; when to consume the six meals is the dieter's personal choice. You can have 3 fuelings in the morning and afternoon then have a "Lean and green" meal in the evening and end the day with 2 fuelings.

Remember, there should be 2-3 hours of the gap between two consecutive meals in a day. Since you will be using more of the fueling and less of the food on this plan, weight loss is quickly achieved using this plan. It is often suggested for the early stage of the lean and green weight loss program because it helps activate the fat burn.

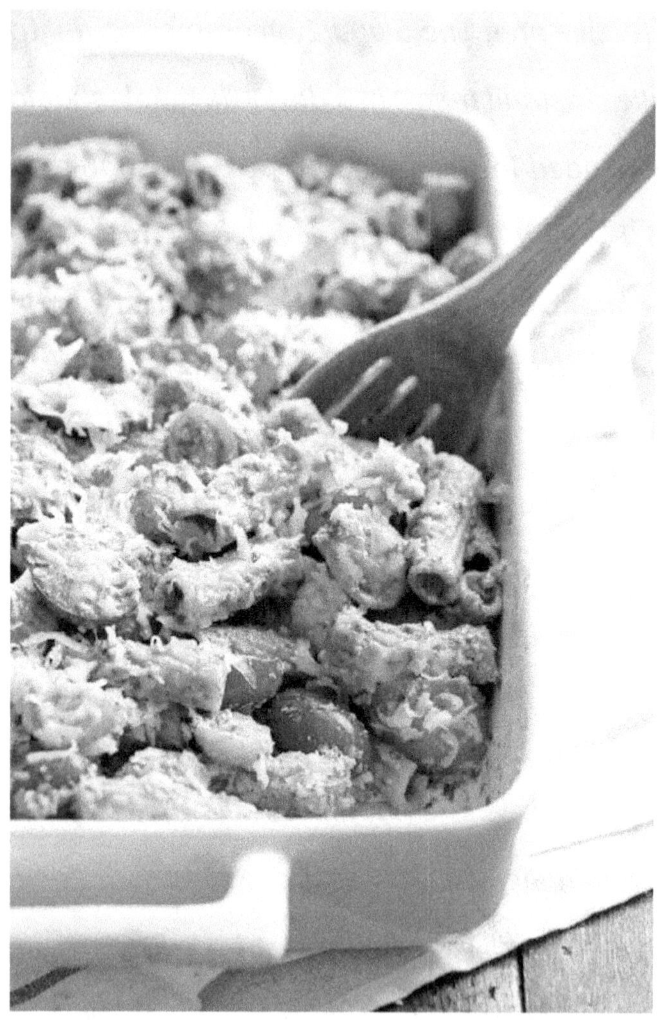

This is the second plan is comparatively easier and simpler than the first plan. This approach recommends the use of 4 fuelings in a day along with 2 lean and green meals and 1 snack. The snack, in this case, should be healthy, and it should be free of carbs and sugars. Sure, this plan is relatively easy, but it does not guarantee quick results. It is overall healthy and can be used as a beginner's approach to starting with.

The 5&1 Plan is the most extraordinary, which includes eating five little dinners each day notwithstanding one "Lean and Green" feast in which you get ready all alone.

Then again, the 4&2&1 Plan is a piece less organized. It accompanies four everyday fueling as well as two of your own "Lean and Green" suppers you make and one Optavia-bought nibble.

GOOD LIFE!

9 781803 612829